30 DAYS TO A HEALTHIER YOU: AN INTRODUCTION TO ALTERNATIVE WEIGHT LOSS TECHNIQUES

TABLE OF CONTENTS

INTRODUCTION

It's common for the road to better physical and mental health to feel like an uphill battle, leaving us discouraged and ready to quit. But do not worry; this book will transform the way you approach weight reduction. We think that getting healthier shouldn't be a difficult, demoralizing task. Instead, it ought to be a motivating and illuminating event that transforms your life in a way that is good and long-lasting. Alternative weight-loss methods can be used in this situation. We will look at a variety of cutting-edge and uncommon weight loss strategies in this manual, emphasizing holistic and doable strategies that fit your particular way of living. We'll explore alternatives to severe diets and strenuous exercise that target the underlying reasons for weight gain and enhance general well-being. You'll find a wealth of information, research-supported insights, and doable steps that will direct you on your transformational journey over the course of the following 30 days. We will examine a variety of ways,

from tried-and-true methods to cutting-edge ideas, such as mindfulness exercises, natural supplements, meals that speed up the metabolism, customized exercise plans, and more. Additionally, our strategy focuses on developing a balanced and healthy relationship between your body and mind, not only in losing weight.

Beyond the scale, adopting alternative weight reduction methods entails adopting a new way of life that boosts energy, boosts confidence, and redefines your total feeling of well-being. Are you prepared to depart

from the traditional approaches to weight reduction
and set out on a journey of empowerment and self-knowledge? If you answered "yes," then let's start on this enlightening trip together. Thank you for visiting "30 Days to a Healthier You: An Introduction to Alternative Weight Loss Techniques. Let's open the doors to a more contented, prosperous, and happy version of yourself!

CHAPTER 1

Examining the Restrictions of Traditional Methods

The quest of obtaining and maintaining a healthy weight has become a common ambition for many people in contemporary culture. Traditional weight loss techniques like diets and exercise have long dominated the weight loss industry. Although these techniques have worked for some people, they have drawbacks that could prevent them from working for others. Investigating alternate weight loss methods that deviate from conventional wisdom is crucial.

A)   Individual Variability

One of the main drawbacks of traditional weight loss techniques is the wide range of responses they elicit from different people. How different bodies consume and store energy depends on their metabolism, genetic makeup, and lifestyle choices. What is successful for one individual may only have marginal effects for another, which may be discouraging and frustrating. In any weight loss journey, individual variability is a crucial factor to take into account. It speaks to the idea that every individual is different and that their unique
genetic, physiological, psychological, and behavioral makeup may have an impact on how they react to weight reduction techniques.

For the purpose of creating individualized and successful weight reduction regimens that take into account each person's unique goals, preferences, and obstacles, it is crucial to recognize and comprehend individual variability.

Individual differences in weight reduction are influenced by a number of factors, including:

- The pace at which an individual's body burns calories and accumulates fat is known as their metabolic rate. While some people may have slower metabolisms that make losing weight more difficult, others may have naturally higher metabolisms that allow them to burn more calories when at rest.

- **Genetics:** Genes can affect a person's body composition, fat distribution, ability to control their hunger, and reaction to various dietary and exercise regimens. The effectiveness with which people lose weight and sustain weight reduction over time may be influenced by genetic predispositions.

- **Hormones:** Imbalances in hormones can affect hunger, appetite, and fat storage. For instance, hormonal abnormalities in the thyroid, leptin, ghrelin, and insulin might impact weight control.

- **Lifestyle:** Personal decisions about one's nutritional preferences, degree of physical activity, sleeping patterns, stress-relieving techniques, and daily routines can have a big impact on how much weight one loses.

- Emotional eating, stress, low self-esteem, and poor mental health are major psychological factors that affect how successfully one loses weight. Due to psychological considerations, some people may find it difficult to manage emotional triggers or stick with weight reduction regimens.

- **Age and gender:** Both of these factors can affect how the body reacts to weight loss attempts. For instance, men tend to have stronger muscle mass and metabolism than women, and age differences in weight reduction may exist.

- **Previous Weight Reduction Attempts:** A person's approach and attitude towards fresh weight reduction efforts might be influenced by past experiences with diets or weight loss attempts.

The significance of individual variation in weight reduction emphasizes the necessity of

tailored strategies to produce fruitful and long-lasting effects. One-size-fits-all or cookie-cutter weight loss plans might not take
into account the particular requirements and difficulties that each person faces. Weight reduction programs may be made more successful and more suited to a person's preferences and capabilities by taking into account individual variations.

Plans for individualized weight loss may include:

- **Comprehensive Assessments:** Conduct in-depth analyses of a person's health, medical background, way of life, food preferences, and level of exercise to pinpoint particular areas that should be improved.
- Setting goals entails working together to establish reasonable, doable targets for weight reduction that are based on personal preferences and health goals.
- Individualized nutrition is the process of creating unique meal plans that take into account a person's food choices, cultural upbringing, and nutritional needs.

- Exercise that is specifically targeted to a person's fitness level, preferences, and objectives while taking into account any physical restrictions or underlying medical issues.

- **Behavioral Support:** Giving people the emotional support they need as well as behavioral techniques
to assist them deal with problems including emotional eating, stress management, and self-motivation.

To sum up, acknowledging and allowing for individual diversity is crucial for effective weight reduction results. Plans for individualized weight loss that take into account certain genetic, physiological, psychological, and lifestyle aspects can provide greater long-lasting effects and enhance general well-being.

Weight loss initiatives may be addressed with better empathy, compassion, and efficacy by embracing the idea of individual diversity.

B)   Plateau Effect

In traditional treatments, calorie consumption is frequently reduced, and physical activity is increased, which results in early weight loss. The body adjusts to these modifications over time, though, and enters a plateau period where weight loss slows down or stops entirely. People may get demotivated and give up on their efforts as a result of this plateau effect.

C)   Yo-Yo Dieting:
Strict diets that severely restrict calories may result in quick weight loss in the short run. However, after the diet is over and usual eating habits return, they might cause a vicious cycle of weight gain. Yo-yo dieting

can be detrimental to metabolic health, in addition to making it difficult to lose weight in the long term.

D)   Effect on the Mind and Emotions

Traditional weight loss techniques can encourage a restricted mentality towards food and body image. An unhealthy relationship with food can develop in a person, which can result in disordered eating habits or

even eating disorders. Furthermore, dissatisfaction over not getting the intended outcomes might result in

emotions of failure and deter people from making additional efforts to lose weight.

Understanding the Advantages of Alternative Approaches:

a) Personalization: Non-traditional weight loss techniques acknowledge the distinctiveness of each person's physique and way of life. These methods frequently use a more individualized strategy, taking into account things like metabolic rate, hormone imbalances, stress levels, and food choices. Non-conventional techniques can provide lasting and successful weight loss strategies by addressing individual requirements.

b) Holistic wellbeing: Non-traditional ways place more emphasis on holistic wellbeing than conventional approaches, which might just pay attention to the physical side of weight loss. They work to foster harmony and general health because they are aware of the connections between physical, mental, and emotional health. This all-encompassing strategy may produce greater long-term results and higher quality of life.

c) Addressing Root Causes: Alternative weight reduction techniques frequently dive deeper into the underlying causes of weight accumulation. They could treat hormonal imbalances, emotional eating triggers, or sleep issues, for instance, that lead to difficulties with weight management. Targeting these root causes can help people lose weight in a way that is more long-lasting.

d) Innovative and Promising Approaches: Non-conventional approaches may include cutting-edge procedures and recent scientific discoveries that go against long-held notions about weight loss. These methods may provide

fresh opportunities for successful weight control and inspire people to try new paths to success.

Changing Attitudes and Adopting Alternative Weight Loss Methods:
a) Letting Go of the "Quick Fix" Mentality:

Alternative approaches to weight management frequently oppose seeking f quick remedies or speedy weight loss. Instead, they place a higher priority on slow, steady growth while emphasizing long-lasting, sustainable changes. This mentality change inspires people to embrace endurance and patience during their weight reduction quest.

b) Embracing Openness to Change:
Investigating different weight reduction methods calls for a flexible mindset. People must be willing to go outside their comfort zones, confront long-held ideas, and think about other viewpoints on weight control.

c) Seeking Professional Advice:
Using unconventional weight loss techniques calls for professional advice. Throughout the process, qualified specialists can offer specialized guidance and assistance, such as licensed dietitians, nutritionists, therapists, or holistic health practitioners.

d) Listening to Their Bodies:
Non-traditional weight reduction techniques frequently place an emphasis on learning to

tune into body cues and to react to individual requirements. Through increased awareness, people can develop healthier relationships with food and exercise, improving their physical and mental health.

As a result, the development of unconventional weight reduction techniques pushes the envelope and promotes a more flexible, individualized, and open-minded approach to obtaining and maintaining a healthy weight. People may start a weight reduction journey that is better suited to their own requirements and circumstances by being aware of the drawbacks of standard procedures and investigating the possible advantages of alternative strategies. To lose weight in a healthy and sustainable way, one must have a thorough awareness of their body as well as a dedication to making long-term, healthy changes.

CHAPTER 2

Intuitive Eating and Mindfulness for Weight Loss

Our connection with food has grown more complex in today's frantic and fast-paced environment. Fad diets' widespread use, social pressures, and continuous exposure to food marketing can cause disordered eating habits and make it difficult to control one's weight.

Promising approaches like mindfulness and intuitive eating urge people to reestablish connections with their bodies, their emotions, and the food they eat. These habits support long-term weight loss and general well-being by encouraging a more mindful and tuned-in approach to eating.

Being present when eating: The Power of Mindful Eating

An age-old method known as mindful eating is based on the Buddhist idea of awareness. Bringing complete consciousness and attention to the current moment while eating is the core of mindful eating. It entails using all the senses to appreciate the tastes, textures, and scents of the meal, as well as actively appreciating the process of feeding the body. The following are the main tenets of mindful eating:

a.) Eating with Full Attention. The practice of mindful eating encourages us to set aside certain times and locations for eating meals, free from interruptions from work or other activities. By doing this, we are able to completely concentrate on the eating process and establish a stronger connection with the meal.

b.) Savoring Each mouthful: Mindful Eating encourages us to slow down and relish each mouthful rather than hurrying through meals. We may get more enjoyment from our meals and know when we are genuinely satiated if we take the time to chew and savor the food completely.

c.) Fostering Gratitude: Mindful eating places an emphasis on being grateful for the food we have and the work that went into making it. The propensity to take food for granted is diminished by this practice, which promotes a more pleasant and conscious connection with eating.

d.) Recognizing Satiety: One of mindful eating's most important advantages is it's capacity to assist us in identifying our bodily cues for hunger and fullness. By closely observing our body's signals, we may more accurately determine when we are truly full and prevent overeating.

Advantages of Mindful Eating for Losing Weight:

- o **Reduced Overeating:** Mindful eating encourages better portion management and prevents overeating by encouraging us to pay attention to our bodies' cues and eat more slowly.

- o **Better Digestion:** When we eat thoughtfully, we take the time to chew each bite fully, which helps with digestion and improves nutrient absorption.

o **Improved Self-Awareness:** Mindful Eating promotes a deeper comprehension of our own eating habits and behaviors, enabling us to make more deliberate and conscientious food decisions.

Intuitive eating advantages for weight loss:

Better Relationship with Food: People may improve their relationship with food by rejecting restrictive diets and embracing intuitive cues, which will lessen the guilt and shame connected to eating.

Sustainable Weight Management: By paying attention to our bodies' hunger and fullness cues, we may manage our weight in a way that is more natural and lasting since we are less likely to go through periods of intense hunger or binge eating.

Body admiration: By emphasizing health and well-being rather than outward looks, intuitive eating encourages body acceptance and admiration. An improvement in one's self-esteem and body image might result from this mental adjustment.

Using Mindfulness Techniques to Combat Emotional Eating

Emotional eating is a common problem in contemporary life. It entails turning to food as a coping method for uncomfortable feelings, stress, or boredom. Using mindfulness practices can help you stop emotional eating:

a.) **Emotional Awareness:** Mindfulness training develops emotional awareness, assisting people in identifying their emotional states and the circumstances that lead to emotional eating. People can create healthier coping mechanisms by being more aware of their emotional responses.

b.) Mindful Coping Strategies: Mindful Eating promotes the investigation of non-food-related coping
techniques rather than using food to dull or divert from emotions. These could include doing deep breathing techniques, writing, or engaging in enjoyable hobbies.

c.) Self-Care Through Mindful Eating: Mindful eating encourages self-compassion and self-care. People may reframe their connection with food and emotional well-being by approaching eating mindfully and treating oneself with respect and empathy. Finally, Mindful Eating and Intuitive Eating are effective weight loss techniques that emphasize self-compassion, mindful awareness, and a balanced perspective on food and eating. A healthy connection with food may be fostered by using mindfulness practices to be present with food, pay attention to the body's cues, and address emotional eating.

This can help people control their weight in a sustainable way and enhance their general well-being. In addition to helping people reach their weight reduction objectives, these practices also encourage the development of a healthy and harmonious relationship between people and their bodies and food.

CHAPTER 3

Holistic Weight Loss Methods

Holistic weight loss solutions have grown in popularity in recent years as individuals look for more all-encompassing and natural ways to reach and maintain a healthy weight. Instead of concentrating only on addressing specific symptoms, these methods emphasize healing the full person—mind, body, and spirit. using herbal remedies and natural supplements, and balancing energy flow through acupuncture and acupressure. Ayurveda and Traditional Chinese Medicine and other ancient practices

a) Ayurveda:

According to Ayurveda, the traditional Indian medical system, maintaining a healthy weight is very important. Unbalances in the doshas, each of which symbolizes various aspects and traits of the body, can lead to weight problems.

The four components of Ayurveda's weight-loss formula

Diet fads and trends encourage a strict diet that may not be healthy for everyone and is sometimes challenging to maintain. This is not the case with Ayurveda's approach to nutrition. Over 5,000 years ago, in what is now India, a kind of complementary and alternative medicine called Ayurveda was developed. It is successful in weight loss because of four factors.

It is Natural: For complete mind-body-spirit well-being, Ayurveda encourages sustained, natural improvements in lifestyle, nutrition, and sleep.

Ayurveda places a strong emphasis on reducing stress through yoga, meditation, medicinal herbs, and purifying treatments.

It is Personalized: It takes into account your needs and promotes self-awareness by stressing that no two people are the same. All three pillars and suggested therapies are given personalized answers.

Health Promotion: Ayurveda empowers the individual, not the sickness. You talk about your family history and personal health objectives during Ayurvedic consultations. Your doctor treats many types of imbalances, including hypothyroidism, obesity, anxiety, and depression, holistically. Consider making these straightforward commitments as well to assist you in achieving your optimum weight:

- **Spend at least three days a week working out.**

The effectiveness of your fitness routine can also be impacted by how and when you exercise. According to Ayurveda, some times of the day are better than others for exercising. These are periods of the day (about 6-10 a.m./p.m.) when atmospheric circumstances provide the system a little bit more vigor and endurance.

Plan your activities during this window in the morning or the evening for the greatest outcomes. Of course, if

such times are inconvenient for you, find a time that does; any exercise is preferable to none.

Ayurveda also advises us to exercise at 50 to 70 percent of our potential, ideally while breathing entirely through our noses. This lessens physiological stress and enables the body to absorb our efforts more fully.

BROWN FAT AND COFFEE FOR WEIGHT LOSS: A SCIENTIFIC RELATIONSHIP

One of the most popular drinks in the world, coffee has long been treasured for its energizing scent and capacity to give a much-needed morning lift. Recent scientific studies have revealed an intriguing link between coffee intake and brown fat activation, beyond its function as an energy booster, perhaps presenting a fresh strategy to promote weight loss attempts.

Brown Fat: The "Good" Fat, Explained:
It's important to first understand brown fat in order to fully appreciate the relevance of coffee's effect on weight reduction. Brown fat has a special function in controlling body temperature and burning calories to produce heat, in contrast to its counterpart, white fat, which stores extra energy and leads to weight gain. It is more abundant in mitochondria, the "powerhouses" of cells that generate energy and give it its distinctive brown color and metabolic capabilities.

Thermogenesis, a process where brown fat burns calories to produce heat, is the main job of brown fat. Researchers from all around the globe have been interested in this energy expenditure since it offers a potential way to fight obesity and promote weight loss objectives.

The Coffee Connection: Beyond Caffeine

Caffeine, a naturally occurring stimulant that is plentiful in coffee beans, is the fundamental component in coffee's ability to aid in weight reduction. It is well known that caffeine speeds up metabolism, increasing energy use and calorie burning. According to studies, caffeine has a potent thermogenic impact that can cause a brief increase in metabolic rate following ingestion.

In addition to caffeine, coffee includes a wide range of bioactive substances, such as trigonelline, quinines, and chlorogenic acid, all of which have been associated with a number of health advantages. These substances may aid in weight control by affecting insulin sensitivity, fat oxidation, and glucose metabolism.

Coffee's Activation of Brown Fat: New Research

Recent studies have examined the connection between coffee intake and brown fat activation, providing exciting new information about the two's possible interactions. According to research in the "Scientific Reports" journal, coffee, in particular, may enhance brown fat activity and boost thermogenesis in people. The scientists discovered that brown fat increased its metabolic activity in response to coffee, which significantly increased calorie expenditure.

The University of Nottingham also used thermal imaging to investigate how coffee affected the activation of brown fat. The scientists noticed that when subjects drank coffee, brown fat was activated, increasing the generation of heat. This implies that coffee's impact on brown fat may go beyond its caffeine level and may also involve other substances found in the drink.

A Comprehensive Approach To Coffee As A Weight Loss Aid

Although the new research on coffee's effect on brown fat activation is encouraging, it's important to think of coffee as a part of a holistic weight reduction plan rather than a miracle cure on its own. A balanced diet, consistent exercise, appropriate hydration, and enough sleep are just a few of the many components of a comprehensive strategy needed for long-term weight loss and general health.

Individual reactions to coffee and its ingredients might also differ. Some people can be more susceptible to the effects of coffee, while others might only notice slight alterations in their metabolism. Additionally, drinking too much coffee might have negative consequences including jitteriness, an elevated heart rate, and irregular sleep patterns.

THE RELATIONSHIP BETWEEN GUT HEALTH AND WEIGHT LOSS: UNTANGLING THE WEB

Often referred to as the "second brain," the human gut is a sophisticated ecosystem made up of many trillions of bacteria, fungi, and other microorganisms that live in the digestive tract. The importance of gut health in many facets of overall well-being, including its impact on weight control, has been highlighted by recent scientific studies. In this article, the intriguing relationship between gut health and weight reduction is explored, emphasizing the ways in which a healthy gut flora might help you lose those excess pounds.

The Diverse World Within the Gut Microbiome: Understanding

The human body and a variety of bacteria called the gut microbiome cohabit together. Numerous biological processes, including digestion, nutrition absorption, and immune system control, depend on this ecosystem. Additionally, it creates necessary vitamins and breaks down certain substances that the body cannot break down on its own.

For sustaining optimum health, the mix of helpful and harmful bacteria in the stomach is essential. Dysbiosis, an imbalance, can cause inflammation, immune system deterioration, and digestive problems. Researchers have recently shown that gut health can affect body weight and metabolic functions

Weight regulation and gut health: The gut-brain axis

The "gut-brain axis," which connects the gut and the brain, is constantly communicating. This network of nerves, hormones, and chemical signals serves as a bidirectional communication system between the stomach and the central nervous system.

The gut-brain axis is influenced by the gut microbiome, and the brain can impact the makeup of the gut microbiota. A healthy gut microbiota can have a good effect on the brain, mood, and cognitive processes. Contrarily, an unbalanced gut flora may result in alterations in appetite, food cravings, and nutrient absorption, which may help to promote weight gain

Energy Production and Gut Health: Caloric Extraction

The ability to extract calories from meals is one way that gut health may influence weight reduction. According to research, an unbalanced gut flora might cause an individual to over-extract calories from food, which increases energy absorption and fat accumulation.

For instance, some bacteria in the gut have the ability to metabolize complex sugars that the human body is unable to perform on its own. The body absorbs more calories as a result of this breakdown, which might result in weight gain. On the other hand, a healthy gut flora may control caloric extraction, promoting more effective energy use and possibly assisting weight loss attempts.

Weight Loss and Inflammation: The Impact of Gut Health

A normal immunological reaction to injury or illness is inflammation. However, persistent inflammation, which is frequently brought on by unbalanced gut flora, can cause a number of health problems, such as insulin resistance and obesity.

Chronic, low-grade inflammation can be caused by an unbalanced gut flora throughout the body. The body's capacity to control hunger and satiety hormones may be hampered by this inflammation, which might result in an increased appetite and overeating. People may have improved appetite control and a stronger sensation of fullness by enhancing gut health and decreasing inflammation, which may help with weight reduction.

Prebiotics and Fiber: Feeding the Gut Microbiome

A fiber and prebiotic-rich diet can help to maintain a balanced gut microbiota. As a prebiotic, fiber feeds the good bacteria in the gut, promoting their growth and maintaining their variety. These healthy bacteria can promote effective digestion, lessen inflammation, and affect weight control as they grow.

Good bacteria's role in weight loss with probiotics

Live beneficial bacteria called probiotics, which are present in some meals and supplements, have grown in popularity due to their potential health advantages. According to some research, some probiotic strains can aid in weight reduction by encouraging healthy gut flora and lowering inflammation. To completely comprehend the connection between probiotics and weight reduction, additional study is necessary.

INTERMITTENT ENERGY RESTRICTION

Cycles of decreased calorie intake and regular calorie intake are part of intermittent energy restriction. It alternates between stages of restriction and maintenance, in contrast to conventional continuous caloric restriction diets, which continually cut daily calorie consumption.

Phase of Caloric Restriction
People consume fewer calories during the Intermittent Energy Restriction's caloric restriction phase than they would normally during the maintenance or regular intake

phases. By consuming fewer calories, you reduce your calorie deficit, which means your body uses more calories than it takes in from meals. As a result, the body starts to utilise fat that has been stored as fuel, which causes weight loss.

Depending on the particular Intermittent Energy Restriction plan and personal preferences, the calorie restriction phase's duration might change. Some people might prefer shorter restrictions, like a few days or a week, while others could prefer lengthier restrictions, like a month. The amount of calorie restriction can also change depending on the individual's age, gender, degree of exercise, and weight loss objectives.

Phase of Maintenance

Following the calorie-restricting phase, people go into the maintenance phase, when they resume their usual calorie intake or one that corresponds to their energy usage.

This interval enables the body to recuperate from the low-calorie period and aids in preventing the metabolic changes brought on by extended caloric restriction.

For several reasons, the maintenance phase is crucial. By giving the body a respite from the calorie deficit, it lowers the risk of nutritional shortages and other metabolic side effects.

The maintenance phase can also aid in preventing the body from going into a condition of constant calorie restriction, which can cause a decrease in metabolism and obstruct long-term weight loss attempts.

Cycle Continues

The recurring cycle of calorie restriction followed by a maintenance period is the fundamental tenet of Intermittent Energy Restriction. For instance, a typical plan would include a cycle of calorie restriction for five days and maintenance eating for the next two days. Alternate-day fasting is a strategy that some diets may employ, in which dieters alternate between days of low-calorie consumption and days of normal eating.

The cycles' duration and frequency can be adjusted based on each person's tastes and objectives. While some would prefer longer cycles, other people could find success with shorter cycles. Individuals may tailor their strategy based on what suits their lifestyle and weight reduction journey the best thanks to IER's flexibility.

Benefits and Intermittent Energy Restriction Mechanisms

Metabolic Flexibility:

The goal of Intermittent Energy Restriction is to encourage metabolic flexibility, or the body's capacity to alternate between using glucose and fat reserves for energy. The body may be trained to effectively use fat as an energy source during the restriction phase and glucose during the maintenance phase with the aid of the alternating caloric restriction and maintenance phases. This adaptation might improve metabolic health overall and boost fat burning under calorie restriction.

Reduced Adaptation: One possible benefit of Intermittent Energy Restriction is its capacity to lessen metabolic adaptation, a condition in which the body responds to calorie restriction by slowing its metabolic rate. Diets that include constant calorie restriction may cause this adaptation, which will make it more difficult to lose weight over time. With this, the intermittent calorie restriction may lessen the degree to which this adaptation occurs, perhaps preserving a greater metabolic rate during the maintenance periods and promoting long-term weight loss.

Sustainability: Because it does not create prolonged deprivation, some people find it more sustainable than typical calorie-restriction diets. The alternate cycles allow for occasional indulgences and may, over time, make sticking to the regimen more tolerable.

Hormonal Regulation: According to certain research, it can have favorable effects on hormones involved in controlling hunger and fat metabolism. For instance, it has been demonstrated that methods that resemble intermittent fasting can affect the hormones leptin and ghrelin, which regulate appetite and fullness. The modulation of these hormones may help with better appetite suppression and maybe support weight reduction.

SPERFOODS FOR WEIGHTLOSS

Moringa: A plant native to South Asia and Africa known as the "miracle tree," moringa is also known as. Its leaves are rich in antioxidants like quercetin and chlorogenic acid as well as vitamins A, C, and E, calcium, iron, and other necessary elements. According to studies, the bioactive ingredients in moringa may help people lose weight. For instance, some animal studies have indicated that moringa extracts can enhance fat metabolism and help people lose weight. More human study is needed to completely confirm these benefits, though. Furthermore, the high fiber content of moringa may aid in promoting satiety and lowering daily calorie consumption.

Black Rice: Black rice, sometimes referred to as forbidden rice, is a historic grain that was originally only offered to Chinese emperors because of its excellent nutritional content. Anthocyanins, potent antioxidants, are what give it its unique black hue. Black rice is a fantastic source of fiber, which promotes a feeling of fullness and helps with digestion as well as appetite management. Because of its low glycemic index, it slowly distributes glucose into the blood, avoiding sudden increases in blood sugar that can trigger cravings and binge eating. In addition, black rice's antioxidants may reduce inflammation, which has been related to obesity and weight gain.

Chia Seeds: Because of their amazing nutritional profile, chia seeds have become well-known as a superfood. They are a great source of fiber, protein, plant-based omega-3 fatty acids, and important minerals including calcium and magnesium. Chia seeds create a gel-like material when they are in touch with fluids, which swells in the stomach and causes a sense of fullness. This satiety effect can aid in controlling appetite and calorie consumption overall. The soluble fiber in chia seeds also facilitates digestion and may enhance intestinal health, both of which are crucial for preserving a healthy weight.

Hemp Seeds: Though they come from the cannabis plant, hemp seeds don't have any psychotropic ingredients. The nine necessary amino acids that the body cannot manufacture on its own are all present in them, making them a rich source of complete protein. A healthy metabolism depends on protein since it supports muscle mass and makes you feel more satisfied. Omega-3 and omega-6 fatty acids, which can help regulate hormones and enhance general well-being, are also abundant in hemp seeds.

Spirulina: A blue-green algae that may have health advantages, spirulina has been ingested for generations. With a wealth of vitamins, minerals, and antioxidants like phycocyanin, it is very nutrient-dense. According to certain research, spirulina may aid in weight loss and lipid profile improvement. It is thought that the protein in spirulina might help people feel fuller longer and help them resist the impulse to overeat. Additionally, its antioxidant capabilities may aid in reducing oxidative stress and inflammation, which are connected to metabolic problems and obesity.

Kelp Noodles: Made from brown seaweed kelp, kelp noodles are a low-calorie substitute for regular spaghetti. They almost entirely lack fat and contain alginate, a soluble fiber that may aid in weight loss. Alginate has been demonstrated to heighten sensations of fullness and postpone stomach emptying, both of which result in lower calorie consumption. Kelp noodles are also gluten-free, making them perfect for people who have a sensitivity to gluten or want to consume less carbs.

Wheatgrass is the young grass of the wheat plant and is a powerhouse of antioxidants, vitamins, and minerals. Wheatgrass is not specifically associated with weight reduction, but its high nutritional content helps improve general health, which is crucial when starting a weight loss journey. Wheatgrass advocates assert that it can speed up metabolism and facilitate detoxification, although there is little scientific data to back up these assertions. However, using wheatgrass in a balanced diet can enhance nutrient uptake and general well-being.

Jerusalem Artichoke: Also known as sunchokes, Jerusalem artichokes are root vegetables that are high in inulin, a soluble fiber. As a prebiotic, inulin encourages the development of healthy gut microbes. More and more experts agree that maintaining a healthy gut flora is crucial for general wellness, including controlling weight. Furthermore, the fiber in Jerusalem artichokes aids in digestion and may induce satiety, which may result in a reduction in calorie consumption.

Amaranth: This ancient grain has a remarkable nutritional profile and is naturally gluten-free. It is a good source of fiber, vitamins, and minerals

as well as protein. Amaranth is a beneficial addition to a diet for losing weight because of its high protein and fiber content, which can aid with promoting a sensation of fullness and lowering appetite. The grain also contains a lot of lysine, an important amino acid that is sometimes deficient in other cereals. Amaranth may be a well-rounded source of nourishment and aid in weight loss when it is included in your meals.

The following are some general recommendations of metabolic-boosting foods:

- Foods that are warm and prepared are preferred over those that are cold and uncooked. Good options include stews, soups, and steamed veggies.
- **Spices:** Incorporate hot spices like ginger, black pepper, cayenne, and mustard seeds into your diet. These can increase metabolism and digestion.
- Foods with bitter and astringent flavors should be consumed since they can assist minimize mucus production and water retention. Leafy greens, turmeric, fenugreek, and dandelion greens are a few examples.

- **Light Fruits:** As opposed to heavier and sweeter fruits like bananas and dates, lighter fruits like apples, pears, and berries are often better for balancing energy.
- **Legumes:** Lentils, mung beans, and split peas are good sources of protein.
- **Honey:** Honey can be used sparingly as a natural sweetener.
- **Herbs:** Some herbs, including Guggulu, punarnava, and trikatu (a blend of ginger, black pepper, and long pepper)

However, it is best to limit or stay away from specific items that might aggravate the system such as:
- Reduce or stay away from dairy items with high-fat content, such as cheese, ice cream, and whole milk.

- Avoid eating too many sweet and heavy fruits, such as bananas, melons, and avocados.
- Consume as little wheat and processed grains as possible.
- Reduce your consumption of fried and fatty meals because they might make you feel heavier and congested.
- Avoid drinking cold drinks and fizzy drinks since they might stifle your digestive fire.

Keep in mind that Ayurveda is a holistic medical system, therefore while adhering to a particular diet, individual constitution, imbalances, and environmental influences should all be taken into consideration. It's always advisable to speak with a certified Ayurvedic practitioner to find out which dietary and lifestyle suggestions are most suited to your individual requirements.

- **Every morning, do fifteen minutes of yoga.**

Body, mind, and soul are all benefited by the extremely potent practice of yoga. It arouses, lubricates, and cleanses the body, stimulates and massages the digestive organs, tones the joints and muscles, boosts circulation ignites the digestive fire and makes detoxification easier.

Yoga also promotes mental and emotional equilibrium, relaxation of the neurological system, and activation of the vital life energy that is inside each of us.

In the end, beginning your day with a few minutes of yoga prepares you for a balanced and productive day, one that is less affected by unneeded tension and harmful appetites and is instead led by clarity, insight, and a natural propensity to honor one's Self and one's body.

- Eat three full meals every day.

A slow metabolism can potentially be made slower by consuming too little. Eating adequately sized meals at reasonable intervals is necessary to effectively stoke the digestive capacity so that the body is not overloaded with the amount of food that needs to be digested or the frequency at which it is consumed.

A crucial balance is achieved by eating three digestible, healthful meals each day without snacking in between. It makes sure that the digestive fire is sufficiently aroused and even helps it get stronger.

Before meals, you can stoke the digestive fire

If you want to go even further, you may stimulate your digestion by chewing a slice of fresh ginger the size of a nickel with a sprinkle of sea salt, a few drops of lime juice, and around 1/4 teaspoon of honey about 30 minutes before lunch and supper.

- Create a daily schedule to help you stick to your obligations.

b) Traditional Chinese Medicine

The idea of energy flow and the harmony of Yin and Yang in the body are related to weight control. It recognizes a number of patterns of discord, such as stagnation or moisture buildup in the body that can lead to weight increase. These imbalances are addressed in order to promote weight reduction through the use of herbal treatments, acupuncture, and dietary modifications. Traditional Chinese Medicine would advise including meals with warming characteristics, for instance, to enhance circulation and lessen stagnation.

USING HERBAL TREATMENTS AND NATURAL SUPPLEMENTS TO INCREASE METABOLISM:

a) Herbal Treatments:

Several plants have been utilized for weight reduction and metabolic assistance throughout history. For instance, green and oolong teas are high in catechins, a substance that may encourage the oxidation of fat.

Another well-known plant, *garcinia cambogia,* is said to reduce hunger and prevent the formation of fat.

b) Natural Supplements: Additions for Weight Loss

It's tempting to search for assistance everywhere when you want to lose weight. When considering dietary supplements or herbal therapies, bear in mind that many of them have received mixed ratings from studies. The claims aren't always well supported by evidence, and some might pose health hazards. Before attempting any, first, speak with your doctor.

Many natural vitamins and herbs are used in traditional Chinese medicine to help weight reduction by

improving digestion, metabolism, and energy balance. Although these supplements have been used for centuries, there hasn't been any scientific study on how helpful they are in promoting weight reduction. Here are some typical Chinese herbal medicines for weight loss:

Hoodia

This particular plant may be found in Africa's Kalahari Desert. The National Center for Complementary and Alternative Medicine states that Bushmen historically utilized the stem of the root to quench their thirst and quench their hunger during protracted hunts. Currently, it is promoted as an appetite suppressor.

P57, a component included in hoodia, is thought to reduce appetite by making you feel satiated. However, there is no solid proof that it is secure or efficient.

7-Keto-DHEA

Your body naturally contains this. By increasing your metabolism and causing you to burn more calories throughout the day, it could aid in weight loss.

In a few short studies, those who took 7-keto-DHEA lost considerably more weight than those who received a placebo (a fake tablet). This was in conjunction with moderate activity and a low-calorie diet.

Green Tea

Due to the abundance of catechins in green tea, especially epigallocatechin gallate (EGCG), it may help in weight reduction. Thermogenesis is accelerated by EGCG, and fat is burned more efficiently, increasing caloric expenditure. Green tea can also increase metabolism and insulin sensitivity, which aids in controlling blood sugar levels and reducing cravings. A small amount of caffeine in it may provide you with an energy boost for exercise. Additionally, green tea has antioxidant qualities that assist general health when trying to lose weight. While not a solo weight-loss strategy, adding green tea alongside a healthy diet and active lifestyle may have some modest advantages.

Ginseng

Due to it's adaptogenic qualities, ginseng, a common plant in traditional Chinese medicine, may indirectly aid in weight loss. It boosts energy levels and aids in the body's adjustment to stress, encouraging movement and general vigor. Ginseng can encourage a more active lifestyle by increasing energy and stamina, which may have positive effects on weight loss. Additionally, ginseng may assist healthier eating choices by helping to control blood sugar levels and lowering the desire for sugary foods.

While ginseng may be a useful supplement, it shouldn't be used in place of a balanced diet and regular exercise

Rhubarb

Rhubarb is recognized for it's therapeutic benefits in addition to it's culinary usage in pies and sweets. *Rheum palmatum* or *Rheum officinale,* the root of the rhubarb plant, is used as an herbal treatment to maintain digestive health and encourage regular bowel movements.

It is a natural laxative that helps to relieve constipation because it's main active ingredients, such as anthraquinones, stimulate the gastrointestinal system.

By aiding digestion and cleansing, rhubarb may help indirectly with weight control attempts by encouraging smoother bowel movements and lowering constipation.

Citrus aurantium

Southeast Asia is the home of the citrus fruit known as *Citrus aurantium*, sometimes referred to as the bitter orange. The fruit's peel (zest) and other parts have been utilized for a variety of therapeutic reasons. Synephrine is a substance found in bitter orange extract, notably from the fruit's peel, and is thought to have stimulant-like effects on the body.

Bitter orange is frequently used to maintain digestive health and improve digestion. It is also thought to enhance general wellness and aid in the relief of some respiratory conditions. Due to it's capacity to boost metabolism and fat breakdown, bitter orange has also been used in weight reduction products.

However, it's vital to use caution while using bitter orange supplements, particularly those that include synephrine, which may have stimulant qualities and may raise blood pressure and heart rate.

Chinese hawthorn

This is a fruit-bearing shrub that is indigenous to China and other regions of Asia. It's scientific name is *Crataegus pinnatifida*, or Shan Zha in Chinese. The fruit and it's accompanying components, such as the
leaves and flowers have been utilized for their therapeutic benefits for generations. Chinese Hawthorn is largely utilized to enhance gastrointestinal health and assist digestion. It is thought to ease bloating and indigestion and aid in the digestion of meals. Flavonoids, procoyanidins, and organic acids are some of the substances in the fruit

that contribute to it's favorable effects on digestion.

Additionally, it is known to have modest diuretic qualities, which might improve overall fluid balance in the body and aid in reducing water retention.

Regarding it's possible involvement in weight management, it is not a supplement for weight reduction in the traditional sense; but, by aiding better digestion, decreasing bloating, and encouraging the excretion of extra fluids, it's digestive and diuretic qualities may indirectly benefit weight management efforts.

Chinese hawthorn is frequently used in a variety of products, such as herbal teas, extracts, and as a component in classic Chinese foods and sweets.

Cinnamon

The inner bark of various tree species in the genus Cinnamomum is the source of the common spice known as cinnamon. Due to it's numerous health advantages, it has been utilized for millennia in traditional medicine, including Ayurveda and traditional Chinese medicine.

It is thought to promote insulin sensitivity and assist control blood sugar levels in connection to weight management. In doing so, it could help people seeking to maintain their weight by helping to curb cravings for sugary foods and carbs. In addition to improving energy levels and decreasing sensations of hunger, stable blood sugar levels also assist overall nutritional management.

Additionally, cinnamon contains anti-inflammatory and antioxidant characteristics that can aid in general health and well-being when trying to lose weight.

Cinnamon is frequently used as a spice in cooking and baking, and it is simple to use in a variety of foods and drinks. But as large amounts of cinnamon pills or extracts may have negative side effects, excessive ingestion should be avoided.

Lotus Leaf

Nelumbo nucifera, usually referred to as lotus leaf, is an aquatic Asian native plant that has been valued for millennia, people have appreciated the lotus plant's leaves for it's medical qualities and for their favorable effects on health. It is said to have diuretic characteristics, which can aid in promoting the body's excess water loss when it comes to weight control. This diuretic action may assist to lessen bloating and water retention while temporarily lowering body weight. Lotus leaf is also known to have astringent qualities that can help tone and tighten tissues. It is frequently used to assist digestion, treat difficulties with diarrhea, and reduce excessive mucus formation. Dietary supplements, herbal extracts, and teas are frequently sold with lotus leaves.

Fucoxanthin

A carotenoid pigment called fucoxanthin is present in brown seaweed like wakame, hijiki, and brown algae. Due to it's possible health advantages, notably in terms of weight control, it has drawn attention recently.

Fucoxanthin may have a number of processes that might aid in attempts to lose weight, according to research. Adipocytes, or fat cells in the body, are one of it's main impacts. It is thought to boost the production of certain proteins that aid in thermogenesis, the process of turning stored fat into energy. In other words, it could encourage the burning of fat, especially in white adipose tissue, which is frequently linked to weight gain. It has been demonstrated that fucoxanthin may have an impact on the liver's metabolism of fat, which may assist to prevent the buildup of fat triglycerides in the liver cells. It may indirectly help with better metabolism and weight management by promoting liver function.

While fucoxanthin exhibits potential as a natural weight-management supplement, additional investigation is required to completely comprehend it's impact on human weight reduction and it's long-term safety profile. Additionally, fucoxanthin is

often used as a dietary supplement rather than as a stand-alone
weight-loss aid. It needs to be combined with a good diet, frequent exercise, and an active lifestyle.

Astragalus

This is a prominent plant that has been used for generations for its different health-promoting characteristics. It's technical name is *Astragalus membranaceus*, or Huang Qi in Chinese. It is regarded as an adaptogenic herb, which means that it boosts general vigor and well-being while assisting the body in adjusting to stress.

It supports the body's life force, which is linked to the immune system's ability to fight off outside diseases.

Astragalus may aid in preventing diseases and infections by boosting the immune system.

Although Astragalus is not often associated with weight reduction, some of it's unintended advantages may help with weight control. For instance, Astragalus may promote physical activity and regular exercise, which are crucial for weight management, by enhancing general energy levels and vitality.

In addition, Astragalus is employed to assist the kidney and spleen functions, all of which are important for metabolism and digestion. Astragalus may aid in the body's effective use of nutrients and assist in improved weight management by encouraging healthy digestion and metabolism.

There are several ways to consume astragalus, including teas, herbal extracts, and nutritional supplements. It is frequently used as remedies to address certain health issues and promote general wellness.

Liu Wei Di Huang Pian

A traditional Chinese herbal compound called Liu Wei Di Huang Wan, also called Liu Wei Di Huang Pian or Six Flavor Rehmanni. It has a lengthy history and is frequently recommended for a wide range of illnesses, especially those that affect the kidney and liver.

Six essential herbs are used in the mixture, including:

Root of Rehmannia (Shu Di Huang)

Fruit of the Corn (Shan Zhu Yu)

Root, Dioscorea (Shan Yao)

Yam in Chinese (Fu Ling)

Zé Xie: Poria Mushroom

Rhizome of alisma (Mu Dan Pi)

The kidney and liver systems are principally nourished and toned by Liu Wei Di Huang

Wan. For general well-being, vitality, and longevity, these organs are crucial. The combination is frequently used for ailments including chronic tiredness, vertigo, lower back discomfort, night sweats, and dry eyes that are caused by kidney and liver abnormalities.

It is not a specific weight reduction treatment when it comes to weight control. Healthy kidney and liver function can improve metabolism, digestion, and general health. Supporting the body's vital energy and balance can help people feel more energised, which may, in turn, help them lead an active lifestyle and exercise frequently, both of which are crucial for weight control.

These formulae are frequently given based on a person's unique patterns of disharmony; the dose and length of usage may change depending on the person's health and reaction to the formula.

Gynostemma

Gynostemma pentaphyllum, sometimes referred to as Gynostemma or Jiaogulan, is a plant that is indigenous to Southeast Asia, including China and Thailand. It belongs to the Cucurbitaceae family, which is also made up of melons and cucumbers. Gynostemma is regarded as an adaptogenic herb in traditional Chinese medicine which means that it aids in the body's ability to cope with stress and fosters general equilibrium and wellbeing. This herb has a long history of usage and it is sometimes known as the "immortality herb" due to it's health advantages and propensity to lengthen life. It is often made as an herbal tonic or drunk as an herbal tea.

It has a number of physiological impacts on the body that may assist with weight loss attempts in an indirect manner. These impacts include, among others:

Metabolism promotion: Gynostemma is believed to improve metabolism, which may help break down fats and carbs and promote weight control.

Increased vitality and energy: Gynostemma may promote increased physical activity and exercise, which are essential for maintaining a healthy weight. Gynostemma, as an adaptogen, can help the body deal with stress more successfully. Reducing stress may indirectly support healthier eating patterns and general well-being. It may aid in controlling blood sugar levels, lessening the desire for sweets, and promoting a healthy diet.

White Mulberry Leaf

The leaf of the white mulberry tree is referred to as *Morus alba* in scientific literature. In traditional medicine, it has a long history of usage, especially in Asian nations like China, Korea, and Japan.

This is a cooling herb that is frequently used to promote different aspects of health. Blood sugar control is one of it's well-known conventional applications. Compounds found in white mulberry leaves, such as 1-deoxynojirimycin (DNJ), may assist to block certain enzymes involved in the digestion of carbohydrates, perhaps resulting in a delayed release of sugar into the circulation. The potential advantages of this trait for those with diabetes or those trying to control their blood sugar levels have generated attention.

The possible impact of white mulberry leaf on blood sugar control in connection to weight management may indirectly assist weight reduction initiatives. It may help reduce cravings for sweet meals and improve appetite management by stabilizing blood sugar levels.

The white mulberry leaf is frequently used in herbal teas, extracts, and conventional herbal preparations.

An overall healthy lifestyle, frequent exercise, and a balanced diet are all necessary for long-term weight management.

Job's Tears

Coix lacryma-jobi, also known as Yi Yi Ren in Chinese, is the scientific name of the grain-bearing plant known as Job's Tears. Due to it's therapeutic qualities, it is frequently used to enhance several areas of health and is regarded as a cooling herb. They are generally recognized for their diuretic effects, which can encourage urine and aid the body in flushing out extra fluids. For people who have water retention and edema, this diuretic action could be helpful. It's diuretic properties may indirectly help with weight management by lowering water retention and bloating.

It's important to understand that any weight loss brought on by diuresis mostly results from a brief decrease in water weight, not fat loss. It nourishes the spleen and stomach, improves digestion, and treats dampness-related diseases in Traditional Chinese Medicine. It can be ingested in a variety of ways, including as an ingredient in conventional herbal preparations, herbal extracts, and herbal teas.

Chinese skullcap

It's scientific name is *Scutellaria baicalensis,* or Huang Qin in Chinese. It is indigenous to Asia, namely China.

It's anti-inflammatory, antioxidant and antibacterial qualities are highly regarded. Chinese skullcap is said to have medical properties due to it's main active ingredients, *baicalin,* and *baicalein.*

Despite not being especially renowned as a weight reduction herb, Chinese skullcap may still indirectly help with weight control due to it's possible anti-inflammatory qualities. It is thought that chronic inflammation contributes to a number of health problems, including obesity and metabolic diseases. Chinese skullcap may promote general health by lowering inflammation, which can help with weight loss plans.

Chinese skullcap has also been researched for it's possible impact on blood sugar management and metabolism. According to some studies, it could improve insulin sensitivity, which is crucial for preserving stable blood sugar levels and lowering the desire for sugary meals. It is sold as dietary supplements, herbal teas, and herbal extracts among other things.

Forsythia

Is a flowering shrub that is indigenous to East Asia, including China and Korea. It's scientific name is *Forsythia suspensa*, and it's Chinese name is Lian Qiao. Due to it's therapeutic qualities, it is frequently used to treat a variety of health issues, especially those connected to heat and inflammation For ailments including fever, sore throat, and respiratory infections, it is frequently recommended.

Even while forsythia isn't primarily renowned as a herb for weight reduction, it's possible anti-inflammatory and antibacterial effects might still indirectly aid in weight control. Obesity and metabolic abnormalities are only two examples of the many health problems that chronic inflammation may cause. It may improve general health by lowering inflammation and boosting the immune system, which may help with weight control. It is said to have detoxifying effects and is used to remove heat and toxins from the body. A body that is balanced and healthy is more likely to support a long-term strategy for weight management. It is frequently utilized as an ingredient in conventional herbal formulations, herbal teas, and herbal extracts.

L-carnitine is a naturally occurring substance that is essential for the body's energy metabolism. It is produced in the liver and kidneys and is a derivative of the amino acids lysine and methionine. The primary function of L-carnitine is to deliver fatty acids to the mitochondria, the powerhouse of the cell, where they are digested and turned into energy.

Small levels of L-carnitine may be found in a variety of meals, particularly in dairy and meat products that come from animals. Additionally, it is advertised as a dietary supplement for enhancing exercise performance and is offered in supplement form.

Due to it's part in fat metabolism, L-carnitine has been said to provide potential advantages in terms of weight control. L-carnitine is thought to boost the use of stored fat for energy by improving the transport of fatty acids into the mitochondria, which may help in weight loss attempts. Though the benefits of L-carnitine on fat oxidation and exercise performance have been studied, the total effects on weight reduction may not be significant.

It's crucial to remember that there is conflicting data on L-carnitine's ability to help people lose weight, and further studies are required before it's usefulness can be conclusively shown. It is not a magic bullet for weight loss on it's own, and it's benefits on weight control may differ from person to person.

In conclusion, L-carnitine should be taken into account as part of a holistic strategy for weight reduction, which includes a balanced diet, frequent physical activity, and general good living choices, even though it may have some potential advantages for weight management and exercise performance.

Garcinia cambogia fruit

The peel of the Southeast Asian native Garcinia cambogia fruit yields a substance called hydroxy citric acid (HCA). The primary component of *garcinia cambogia*

extract is HCA, which has grown in popularity as a dietary supplement for weight loss.
HCA is thought to have a number of possible weight-loss benefits, including:

Citrate lyase, an enzyme that is involved in the transformation of carbohydrates into fat, is hypothesized to be inhibited by HCA. By inhibiting this enzyme, HCA may lessen the conversion of surplus
carbs into stored fat, which may result in a reduction in fat deposition.
Serotonin levels in the brain, which affect appetite and food desires, may be affected by HCA, according to some research. It is thought that higher serotonin levels
may cause an appetite reduction, aiding with calorie restriction.

Fat Metabolism: It has been hypothesized that HCA supports fat metabolism by encouraging the use of body fat that has been stored as energy, potentially resulting in more fat being burned while exercising. However, there is conflicting information about the efficacy of HCA for managing weight, and the studies' findings have not been definitive. While some studies indicate that it may have only a slight impact on weight

loss, other studies find no discernible difference between it and a placebo.

The HCA in garcinia cambogia extract may have some possible impacts on weight management, but it shouldn't be depended upon as the only way to lose weight. A balanced diet, consistent exercise, a generally

good living choices are all necessary for long-term weight management.

Polygonum multiflorum, also known as **He Shou Wu** or Fo-Ti, for millennia due to it's many health advantages.

He Shou Wu is a Chinese herbal remedy made from the roots of the *Polygonum multiflorum* plant. It is a well-liked tonic herb and highly regarded for it's revitalizing and life-extending qualities.

The plant has the moniker Mr. He in honor of a fable about an elderly man who, after consistently taking the herb, purportedly recovered his young vigor and black hair.

He Shou Wu is generally used to nourish and detoxify the liver and kidneys. The liver and kidneys are regarded as key organs for general health, and it is thought that keeping them in balance is critical for preserving vitality and well-being. Premature graying of hair, weak knees and lower back, and exhaustion are all symptoms associated with kidney and liver abnormalities that are frequently treated with He Shou Wu. When the liver and kidneys are balanced and performing at their best, it can boost general well-being and vitality, which may tangentially benefit weight management attempts by promoting a more active lifestyle. It can be found in a variety of forms, such as herbal teas, extracts, and traditional herbal preparations.

Atractylodes

It's scientific name is *Atractylodes lancea*, called Bai Zhu in Chinese. It is a native of East Asia and is in the same family as sunflowers and daisies. This is regarded as a warming herb and it is frequently used to detoxify the stomach and spleen. The spleen and stomach are thought to be crucial for proper digestion and the creation of general energy. Atractylodes is said to enhance

digestion, boost energy, and advance general health by supporting these organs. It is typically used for spleen and stomach deficiency-related symptoms
like low appetite, exhaustion, and loose stools. Additionally, it is thought to have diuretic qualities that might encourage urine and lessen water retention.
Additionally, due to it's diuretic effects, it could be possible to temporarily lower body weight by reducing bloating and water retention.
Common applications for atractylodes include herbal teas, herbal extracts, and traditional herbal preparations.
This herb may have some possible health advantages, but it is not a stand-alone weight-loss method. A balanced diet, consistent exercise, and a healthy lifestyle are necessary for long-term weight

management. This can be a beneficial supplement to a general health and wellness program, especially for people looking for assistance with their energy and digestion, but it shouldn't be the only thing they use to lose weight.

Sophora flower

The blossom of the Sophora japonica tree, which is indigenous to East Asia, is known as the Sophora flower, also known as Flos Sophorae and Huai Hua in Chinese. This flower is a traditional remedy for diseases linked to heat and moisture in the body and is regarded as a cooling herb. The liver and intestines are two places where it's frequently recommended to remove heat and lower inflammation.

Traditional uses of the sophora flower include promoting normal blood flow and treating problems with blood stagnation including bruising, bleeding, and irregular menstruation. Since enhanced circulation is crucial for the smooth operation of the body's systems, it's capacity to promote blood circulation may have some indirect advantages for general health.

The body may promote general well-being and vitality when it is in balance and free of excess heat and moisture, which may indirectly help weight management efforts by promoting a more active lifestyle. This flower is frequently used in herbal teas, herbal extracts, and conventional herbal preparations.

Based on your unique health situation, requirements, and potential interactions with other drugs or therapies, they can assist in choosing the supplements that are most suitable for you. Additionally, it's critical to keep in mind that supplements by themselves are not a foolproof way to lose weight; rather, a comprehensive strategy that incorporates a balanced diet and regular exercise which is necessary for reaching and maintaining a healthy weight.

Acupuncture and acupressure are two methods for balancing the body's flow

a) Acupuncture

Acupuncture is a traditional Chinese medicine technique that includes inserting tiny needles into certain body sites. Acupuncturists may focus on points associated with digestion, hunger control, and stress reduction in order to aid with weight loss. By reducing cravings, enhancing digestion, and enhancing general well-being, acupuncture may aid in more efficient weight control. Traditional Chinese medicine's old treatment method of acupuncture has gained popularity for it's ability to support weight control initiatives.

Acupuncture, which takes a holistic approach to health, concentrates on balancing the body's flow by stimulating particular acupoints. The method provides a special combination of advantages that support long-term weight loss and enhanced general well-being.

By **controlling hunger and appetite,** acupuncture is one of the main ways it helps people lose weight. The hormone ghrelin, which increases hunger, can be released less often by activating acupoints. Acupuncture can simultaneously improve leptin sensitivity, which signals fullness and improves appetite control, and reduces cravings for harmful foods. Additionally, acupuncture has several advantages for weight loss, including reducing stress. Emotional eating, which occurs when people turn to food for

solace when under stress, is common.
Acupuncture encourages the body's natural
mood enhancers, endorphins, to be released,
which lowers stress levels and lessens the
propensity to overeat.

Acupuncture helps **enhance digestion and
metabolism**, two important aspects of
weight management. Acupuncture aids the
body's effective digestion and thyroid
function, which prevents food from being
stored as fat and allows it to be converted
into energy. These treatments boost blood
circulation, which promotes nutrient
absorption and waste disposal, further
enhancing the body's capacity to absorb
nutrients.

The **balance of hormones** is yet another
important way that acupuncture aids in
weight loss. Particularly in women,

hormonal abnormalities involving insulin, cortisol, and estrogen can cause weight gain. By balancing these hormones, acupuncture promotes weight reduction by fostering a more tranquil interior environment.

Acupuncturists frequently talk with their patients about lifestyle concerns during treatments. This covers things like eating habits, exercise routines, and sleeping habits.

Acupuncturists provide continuing support throughout the process and provide advice on how to make better decisions and create reasonable weight reduction goals.

Despite the fact that acupuncture has several advantages for weight reduction, it is important to understand that it cannot be used as a stand-alone treatment. Instead, it works best when used in a complete weight-management plan. A balanced diet and moderate exercise in addition to acupuncture can produce more significant and long-lasting improvements. Additionally, while using acupuncture for weight reduction, individual variances should be taken into consideration. Because every person's body and health profile are different, individualized acupuncture treatment programs that are catered to each person's requirements and objectives are necessary. When starting a weight reduction program based on acupuncture, it is also essential to seek the advice of a licensed acupuncturist or healthcare provider.

Acupuncturists will perform a complete evaluation of the client's health and lifestyle, taking into account any underlying medical issues that can affect weight reduction. As a result, acupuncture provides a multimodal strategy for weight reduction, addressing both the physical and mental aspects that affect one's path toward weight control.

Acupuncture aids in long-term weight loss and enhanced general health by regulating hunger, reducing stress, enhancing digestion and metabolism, balancing hormones, and offering lifestyle advice. People can maximize the effectiveness of acupuncture in helping them lose weight by combining it with a healthy diet and regular exercise.

b) Acupressure

Acupressure uses a similar approach to acupuncture, but instead of inserting needles, it applies pressure to certain locations. Self-acupressure is an option, as is consulting a qualified practitioner for advice.

Acupressure works to stimulate these areas in order to encourage the flow of energy and assist with weight loss goals.

CHAPTER 4

Functional Movement and Exercise

Many people are turning to functional exercise and movement practices in their search for greater physical fitness and overall well-being. With an emphasis on strength, flexibility, mobility, and stress reduction, these alternative techniques go beyond regular gym workouts and provide a comprehensive approach to fitness. People may improve their fitness journey and attain a more balanced and long-lasting approach to weight control by investigating alternative exercise techniques like Pilates, Yoga, and Dance, participating in functional training, and embracing mind-body activities.

Investigating other forms of exercise such as Pilates, Yoga, and dance

a) Pilates:

Created by Joseph Pilates, Pilates is a low-impact workout technique that emphasizes flexibility, body awareness, and core strength. Pilates routines incorporate regulated motions that focus on the back and abdomen's deep stabilizing muscles. It places a major emphasis on appropriate alignment and breath
control, which helps to build a strong and stable core and enhances body awareness and posture.

b) Yoga: Yoga is an age-old discipline that combines breathing exercises, physical postures, and meditation to enhance one's physical, mental, and spiritual well-being. Yoga comes in a variety of forms, from calming and restorative to vigorous and demanding. It improves power, flexibility, balance, and awareness, making it a great addition to weight-loss initiatives.

c) Dance: Dance is a fun and expressive art form that is also a great way to exercise. Exercises that involve dance, such as ballet, hip-hop, salsa, or modern dance, can enhance muscular tone, cardiovascular fitness, and coordination. A workout regimen may be made more enjoyable and creative by including dance.
Strength, flexibility, and mobility are all improved through functional training.

Exercise techniques known as **"functional training"** place an emphasis on movements that simulate daily activities and enhance functional fitness. Functional workouts work numerous muscle groups concurrently rather than just one at a time.

Techniques for functional mobility and exercise can help with weight loss and general fitness. These workouts can help you lose weight, strengthen your muscles, and enhance your cardiovascular health. Here are some exercises and functional mobility strategies that might help you lose weight:

Weight-Bearing Exercises

Push-ups: This popular workout works the shoulders, triceps, and chest while also involving the core. Push-ups are a strong-building activity that doesn't require any special equipment because your body weight acts as resistance while you complete them.

Squats: The glutes, quadriceps, and hamstrings are largely worked during squats. For stability, they also use their lower back and core muscles. Squats are extremely effective for daily tasks since they imitate the motions of sitting and standing.

Lunges: Lunges are great for working the glutes, hamstrings, and quadriceps in the legs. They are a beneficial workout for total mobility since they help increase balance and stability.

Planks: Planks target the core muscles, which include
the lower back, obliques, and abdominals. They aid in enhancing posture, stability, and core strength, all of which are essential for a variety of athletic activities.

Workouts for The Heart
Running or jogging: Running or jogging is a very efficient strategy to lose weight and strengthen your
heart. It works a variety of muscles and may be performed outside or on a treadmill.

Cycling: Cycling is a low-impact activity that is easy on the joints and gives the heart a great workout. Cycling outside or on a stationary bike helps burn calories and strengthens the legs.

Jump Rope: A quick and effective approach to raising your heart rate is to jump rope. It's an excellent choice for a high-intensity cardio workout and is simple to work into your schedule.

Swimming: Swimming is a total-body workout that is easy on the joints and trains a variety of muscle groups. It can increase flexibility generally, increase endurance, and burn calories.

HIIT (High-Intensity Interval Training)

HIIT incorporates short bursts of intense activity followed by rest intervals. This strategy has been demonstrated to be successful in raising metabolic rate after exercise and burning more calories in less time.

HIIT may be customized to fit individual interests, such as incorporating aerobic workouts like sprinting or cycling with body-weight exercises like burpees, jumping jacks, and mountain climbers.

Functional Education

Functional exercises are of great advantage for enhancing everyday functionality and lowering the risk of accidents because they concentrate on motions that replicate real-life tasks.

Exercising using a medicine ball improves rotational strength, which is essential for many sports and motions.

Step-ups work the glutes and legs while enhancing stability and balance, which are crucial for activities like trekking and stair climbing.

Exercise Circuits

Exercises are performed in a series during a circuit workout with little breaks in between.

It maintains an elevated heart rate, increases calorie burn, and provides cardiovascular advantages.

By mixing several workouts, including bodyweight movements, aerobic exercises, and resistance exercises, you may make a circuit.

Strength Training

To target particular muscle areas during resistance training, external weights like dumbbells, resistance bands, or machines are used.

Resistance exercise can raise your resting metabolic rate and increase muscle mass, which will result in more calories being expended throughout the day.

Exercises using a Swiss ball

By adding a degree of instability to workouts using a stability ball (Swiss ball), you can work more muscles and enhance your balance and coordination.
Swiss ball workouts can involve a variety of motions including ball squats, ball bridges, and ball rollouts, all of which promote weight loss by challenging specific muscle groups.

In conclusion, functional mobility and exercise techniques provide a comprehensive strategy for managing weight and promoting general well-being. People will improve their physical fitness, lower their stress levels, and develop a stronger mind-body connection by exploring alternative forms of exercise like Pilates, Yoga, and Dance, participating in functional training, and embracing mind-body practices. These behaviors enhance long-term health and vitality by aiding in weight control as well as a more balanced and sustainable way of living. As with any fitness regimen, it's crucial to pay attention to your body, make small, incremental advancements, and, as necessary, get advice from trained instructors or medical specialists.

CHAPTER 5

The Influence of Support and Community

Starting a weight loss journey may be a life-changing and occasionally difficult affair. When it comes to giving people the drive, inspiration, and tools they need to effectively lose weight, the power of community and support is vital. Individuals may improve their mental and emotional well-being while cultivating a feeling of belonging and empowerment throughout their weight loss journey by developing a supportive network, taking part in group wellness programs and challenges, and practicing self-care.

Creating a Community of Encouragement and Accountability

An individual's weight loss journey might be positively impacted by developing a supporting network of friends, family, or like-minded people. These people can cheer you on, acknowledge your accomplishments, and inspire you when things become tough. Sharing successes and setbacks with a supportive network fosters responsibility because it encourages people to stick with their objectives. It also gives a place to freely communicate ideas and emotions, encouraging closer relationships with those who have the same understanding and experiences.

Group wellness initiatives and difficulties
Taking part in group health challenges and programs may be a fun and successful method to lose weight. Being a part of a group with the same goals can motivate people to stretch themselves and achieve new heights. Fitness courses and group workouts not only offer social connection

but also the advantages of group motivation and friendly rivalry. Group challenges like step counts, healthy eating targets, or fitness challenges may foster camaraderie and a shared interest in wellness.

Self-care Activities that Promote Mental and Emotional Wellness

Along with physical changes, losing weight demands both mental and emotional toughness. Self-care activities may have a big influence on someone's mental and emotional health while they're being done: Meditation and mindfulness exercises can help people with their stress, anxiety, and emotional eating habits. These techniques help people become more self-aware, which makes it possible for them to react to emotional triggers more logically and compassionately.

Weight control can benefit from stress management strategies such as relaxation exercises, hobbies, or time spent in nature. High-stress levels might trigger emotional eating and impede the process of losing weight.

Prioritizing adequate rest and sleep is crucial for maintaining overall health and well-being. A successful weight loss program depends on hormonal balance, hunger control, and energy levels, all of which are supported by quality sleep.

Self-talk and visualization exercises can help one feel more confident and more certain that they can succeed in their weight reduction objectives. A more upbeat and motivated mentality may be developed through visualizing success and favorable results.

Community and support are advantageous for weight loss.

Increased Motivation: Being a member of a group that is encouraging gives people the drive to continue making progress in losing weight, especially when things are difficult.

Shared Experiences: Creating a strong support system enables people to talk about their struggles, victories, and experiences with others, which promotes a sense of community and understanding.

Responsibility: Support groups provide a certain amount of responsibility, assisting people in adhering to their commitments and aspirations.

Emotional Well-Being: Social interaction in a comforting setting helps lessen emotions of loneliness, tension, and anxiety, which promotes general mental and emotional health.

In conclusion, community and support are hugely important for effective and long-lasting weight loss. Creating a strong support system, taking part in group wellness challenges and programs, and practicing self-care can provide people the inspiration, accountability, and emotional support they need to get over problems and remain dedicated to their weight loss journeys. Accepting the power and inspiration provided by a caring group may result in not just successful weight reduction but also a general feeling of contentment and well-being. People may make their weight loss journey a transforming and inspiring experience by encouraging relationships with others and taking care of their mental and emotional health.

28 DAYS WORKOUT ROUTINE (VARIETIES)

WEEK 1:

Day 1: Yoga Flow (30 minutes) - Start the week with a gentle yoga flow to improve flexibility, reduce stress, and promote mind-body awareness.

Day 2: Bodyweight Circuit (20 minutes) - Perform a circuit of bodyweight exercises, such as squats, push-ups, lunges, and planks, to engage multiple muscle groups and boost metabolism.

Day 3: Tai Chi (20 minutes) - Try a tai chi session to improve balance, reduce tension, and enhance overall body awareness.

Day 4: Rest Day - Allow your body to recover and prepare for the upcoming workouts.

Day 5: Hiking (60 minutes) - Enjoy nature while engaging in moderate-intensity hiking to burn calories and strengthen your lower body.

Day 6: Pilates (30 minutes) - Focus on core strength, stability, and flexibility with a Pilates workout.

Day 7: Dance Cardio (30 minutes) - Have fun with a dance-based cardio workout to elevate your heart rate and burn extra calories.

WEEK 2:

Day 8: Resistance Band Training (25 minutes) - Incorporate resistance band exercises for full-body strength training and toning.

Day 9: Qigong (20 minutes) - Try a Qigong session to improve energy flow, reduce stress, and promote relaxation.

Day 10: Cycling (45 minutes) - Go for a bike ride to work on cardiovascular endurance and lower body strength.

Day 11: Rest Day

Day 12: Swimming (30 minutes) - Head to the pool for a low-impact, full-body workout that burns calories and improves cardiovascular fitness.

Day 13: Yoga (30 minutes) - Focus on holding poses in a yoga practice to build strength and enhance flexibility.

Day 14: Jump Rope (15 minutes) - Jump rope for a quick and effective cardio workout that targets the entire body.

WEEK 3:

Day 15: Kettlebell Workout (25 minutes) - Use kettlebells for dynamic, total-body exercises that boost metabolism and strengthen muscles.

Day 16: Meditation and Breathwork (15 minutes) - Incorporate meditation and breathwork to reduce stress and improve mindfulness.

Day 17: Indoor Climbing (60 minutes) - Try indoor climbing for a fun and challenging full-body workout.

Day 18: Rest Day
Day 19: Aerial Yoga (30 minutes) - Experience the benefits of aerial yoga, which combines traditional yoga poses with the support of a hammock.

Day 20: Rowing (20 minutes) - Use a rowing machine for a low-impact, full-body cardio workout.

Day 21: Barre Workout (30 minutes) - Enjoy a barre workout that combines elements of ballet, Pilates, and strength training for a sculpted physique.

WEEK 4:

Day 22: Hiking or Nature Walk (60 minutes) - Get back outside for another hiking or nature walk session.

Day 23: Restorative Yoga (20 minutes) - Practice restorative yoga to promote relaxation and recovery.

Day 24: Boxing or Kickboxing (30 minutes) - Try a boxing or kickboxing workout for an intense cardio session and stress relief.

Day 25: Rest Day

Day 26: Functional Training (25 minutes) - Focus on functional movements that mimic everyday activities and improve overall strength and mobility.

Day 27: Beach Volleyball (45 minutes) - Engage in a fun game of beach volleyball for a full-body workout.

Day 28: HIIT (High-Intensity Interval Training) (20 minutes) - Finish the month with a high-intensity interval training session for maximum calorie burn and cardiovascular fitness.

Note: Remember to warm up before each workout and cool down afterward. Listen to your body, modify exercises as needed, and always consult with a healthcare professional before starting a new exercise routine, especially if you have any underlying health conditions.
All these must not be fully done but it gives an idea about the varieties of different exercises to do. Enjoy the variety of

exercises and have fun with this alternative 28-day exercise routine for weight loss!